BOOK SUMMARY

LEADING WELL FROM WITHIN

A Neuroscience and Mindfulness-Based
Framework for Conscious Leadership

DANIEL FRIEDLAND, MD

SuperSmartHealth®

Published by SuperSmartHealth Publishing.

ISBN: 978-0-9978538-1-0

SuperSmartHealth
P.O. Box 910286
San Diego, CA 92191-0286
United States of America
Telephone: 858.481.2393
E-mail: Support@SuperSmartHealth.com

For Sue, Zach and Dyl

Table of Contents

Preface

As a busy leader, your time is very valuable. I wrote *Leading Well from Within* to help you make the most of your time, showing you how to first reduce your reactivity when it does more harm than good, and then *leverage* your stress energy into high-performing states of creativity, so you can more fully live your most meaningful life.

I also realize the investment required to tackle a 300-plus-page book can be daunting! So I've created this book summary of *Leading Well from Within* to help you absorb its key concepts and action steps in one sitting.

My hope is that you will use this summary to experience some actionable "aha" moments to show you how valuable a Conscious Leadership mindset can be.

But even more, I hope it will inspire you to immerse yourself in the book, using this summary as a companion, to master the shift from reactivity to creativity in any circumstance.

This skill alone will put you in the top echelon of high-performance leaders, allowing you to shift from success to significance as you transform yourself, your business, your family, your community, and even the world!

The Case for Conscious Leadership

During my crisis of leadership [pages 1–7], you may have noticed a movement between two polarities:

1. *One involves a **reactive mindset**, where we feel threatened with fear, stress, self-doubt, ego, and conflict; where an unconscious and reflexive series of protective responses can dominate our psyche and ripple through our actions, activating similar experiences in others that can instantly drain energy and fragment teams as well as families.*

2. *The other involves a **creative mindset**, where with conscious awareness, self-compassion, and courage, we can lean in and grow, even in our most challenging circumstances. Inspiration, energy, and empathy are present, and innovation can flourish, enabling a team to work well together with transparency and trust and become aligned in a shared vision to more fully focus its collective energy to serve others and something larger than themselves.*

Leaders, and their ability to be aware of and navigate stress, uncertainty, and self-doubt in any given situation, can profoundly influence which mindset dominates.

Introduction, page 8

Before we can lead well in the world, we first need to learn how to lead well from within. *Leading Well from Within* helps you develop the awareness, skills, and practices to engage stress, uncertainty, and self-doubt, and focus on what matters most in life. In other words, it helps you become a more Conscious Leader.

We all experience stress and self-doubt, and we know all too well how it can undermine our performance, our relationships, and even our health. At the same time, we've also experienced moments of high performance, fueled by creativity, proactivity, and a sense of "flow." Whether you're a business leader, healthcare provider, entrepreneur, coach, or parent, you probably want to know: how can I spend less time mired in stress and self-doubt, and more time performing at my peak and feeling inspired, energized, alive, effective, and in the flow?

The truth is that stress can fuel *both* low performance and high performance—and the key is your *mindset*. So I begin the introduction with a story about my own crisis of leadership to reveal two key leadership mindsets:

1. A *reactive mindset*, where stress and self-doubt can cause you to spiral downward into a low-performance state

2. A *creative mindset*, in which you can *leverage your stress energy as an asset* to shift into a high-performance state

I also briefly introduce the 4 in 4 Framework™, a practical process to help anyone make the shift from reactivity to creativity, regardless of the amount of stress you're under in the moment. Instead of just learning how to manage stress, you will learn how to leverage it as creative fuel to achieve even higher levels of performance than you would without any stress at all!

The introduction ends by sharing a roadmap for the book:

Part 1 provides a four-layered foundation of the 4 in 4 Framework: (1) the bottom-line evidence for why it's so crucial for leaders to cultivate a creative mindset today, (2) the brain science behind reactivity and creativity, (3) the key practice of mindfulness, and (4) an overview of the 4 in 4 Framework itself.

Part 2 takes you through each of the four steps of the 4 in 4 Framework to lead well from within. You will learn the specific neuroscience- and mindfulness-based skills and practices you can use right now to leverage your own stress and self-doubt to shift from a reactive to a creative mindset and experience greater health and vitality, deeper relationships, and a greater sense of meaning and fulfillment at work and at home.

Part 3 explains how to apply the 4 in 4 Framework to lead well in the world. You'll learn how to cultivate creativity in your relationships and create thriving cultures within organizations, families, and communities.

Finally, the **conclusion** summarizes the 4 in 4 Framework into one simple step that includes all the others and offers support for lifelong practice and transformation.

Stress and self-doubt are not only normal; they can be potent assets for both *discovering* and *fueling* your most meaningful life. The 4 in 4 Framework will show you how—not just for yourself, but for those you serve.

So let's dive in!

Part 1

The Foundation for
Engaging Conscious Leadership

CHAPTER 1

Evidence and Inspiration for Engaging Conscious Leadership

The skills and practices that allow us to shift from a reactive to a creative mindset, or stay in a creative mindset under pressure, have never been more crucial, since the circumstances and stress we face today feel more threatening than ever. . . .

Research shows that high-performance leadership is indeed correlated with a creative mindset and low-performance leadership with a reactive mindset.

Chapter 1, page 28

Take a moment to bring to mind the most inspiring leader you know. What kind of qualities did that person have—and what qualities did he or she engender in you?

Now, bring to mind the worst leader you've ever encountered. What qualities did that person have—and engender in you?

For most people, the difference is clear. Research shows that the difference between the two boils down to that leader's mindset: a **reactive mindset** diminishes leadership performance, organizational effectiveness, and resiliency against burnout, while a **creative mindset (or Conscious Leadership)** improves them. And the approach of Conscious Leadership is equally effective across industries, from business to healthcare to life at home and beyond.

Chapter 1 lays the first foundational layer of leading well from within: the evidence for how vitally important it is to cultivate Conscious Leadership in business, healthcare, and all other leadership contexts, including parenting, teaching, coaching, and healing others.

9

And it doesn't just enhance your leadership; it's also crucial for preventing burnout and building resiliency, so you can thrive in today's high-stress, high-stakes environment.

Key Points

- According to my experience working with clients, most people define **high-performance leaders** as those who
  - ➤ have vision and purpose
  - ➤ are strategically focused
  - ➤ are decisive and get things done
  - ➤ care about and relate well to people
  - ➤ are humble and compassionate
  - ➤ are courageous and have integrity
  - ➤ are emotionally intelligent
  - ➤ can see the big picture
  - ➤ are highly passionate and innovative
  - ➤ lead from their highest selves
  - ➤ are in service of something larger than themselves
- In contrast, **low-performance leaders** are defined as those who
  - ➤ tend to lead with ego and intimidation
  - ➤ are territorial
  - ➤ micromanage
  - ➤ judge
  - ➤ criticize and blame others
  - ➤ may be wishy-washy and expedient
  - ➤ are emotionally labile and cannot be trusted
  - ➤ may fight for power and control to prove their self-worth, or alternatively take flight from their responsibility or what personally threatens them
  - ➤ lead from ego in service of themselves

- According to the Leadership Circle, a leading organization in leadership assessment, leaders with a **creative mindset** have the abovementioned high-performance qualities. They relate well to people, are authentic, are both systems aware and self-aware, and are achievement oriented. Leaders with a **reactive mindset** have the low-performance qualities. They focus on protecting their ego with a stance of being overly compliant, protective, or controlling.

- According to an IBM study, CEOs named **creativity** as the top quality leaders need to navigate our increasingly complex business environment. In this context, and for the purposes of this book, creativity means not just innovative thinking, but having a greater awareness of yourself, others, and the system in which you operate; connecting authentically and well with others; and achieving meaningful results. This definition may be more akin to *proactivity*: using our knowledge and creativity to anticipate situations and seizing them as opportunities to affect the outcome.

- The Leadership Circle's research shows both a clear correlation between a creative mindset and high-performance leadership, and between a reactive mindset and low-performance leadership on key business outcomes such as new product development, the quality of products and services, sales, revenue growth, market share, and profitability.

- The reactive and creative mindset also impacts burnout and resiliency. In today's high-stress, quickly changing society, 96 percent of senior leaders in business report some degree of burnout, and one-third describe it as extreme. In healthcare, more than 50 percent of physicians experience symptoms of burnout.

- **Burnout** is an ominous triad of symptoms in which individuals experience (1) emotional exhaustion, (2) feel disconnected in their relationships, and (3) experience a reduced sense of personal accomplishment in their work.

- Dealing with burnout is not only debilitating for the leader, but the leader's stress and reactivity can ripple through an organization, eroding the culture and significantly impacting employee engagement and the bottom line.

- Cutting-edge stress research also shows that the harmful effects of stress have a lot to do with your **mindset about stress**: whether you view it as harmful or helpful. For example, a large body of research tells us just how dangerous stress is for our health—yet if you become more stressed about being stressed, it can intensify your reactive mindset and make the problem worse!

- Conscious Leaders are not only high-performance leaders. They also embody the antithesis of burnout. They know how to thrive under stress and engage it with a creative mindset in alignment with their vision and purpose to exude passion and vitality. Even in the most challenging of circumstances, they are able to connect with and inspire others and take all stakeholders into account. And they experience fulfillment and significance in knowing they are serving and contributing value to the greater good. These qualities not only transform the leader, but all they serve—whether a CEO or manager, healer, parent, teacher, coach, spouse, or anyone wanting to contribute more fully to the lives of others.

- The integration of the two worlds of business and healthcare provide a powerful paradigm for developing high-performance Conscious Leadership.

  - ➤ In the **world of business**, the Conscious Capitalism movement provides an inspiring example of how a creative mindset can transform businesses. Its four key values are: (1) Higher Purpose, (2) Stakeholder Orientation, (3) Conscious Leadership, or inspired leadership, where you lead from your highest self in service of something larger than yourself, and (4) Conscious Culture, where leaders, employees, and all stakeholders consciously and actively engage in the communication and collective action that embodies the principles and values of the company and thus allows it to manifest its purpose.

  - ➤ In the **world of healthcare**, the approach of integrative health offers inspiration for the development of Conscious Leadership. Integrative health is a paradigm of healthcare based on "wholeness," which is the origin of the word, "health" itself. The Academy of Integrative Health and Medicine defines "optimal health" as "the conscious pursuit of the highest level of functioning and balance of the physical, environmental, mental, emotional, social, and spiritual aspects of human experience, resulting in a dynamic state of being fully alive."

- Much of the philosophy of Conscious Capitalism and integrative healthcare integrated within this book leads to the development of conscious, high-performance leaders—i.e., healthy leaders who can create healthy organizations, families, and communities, which thrive and make a meaningful difference in the lives of others.

Learn How Your Brain Works to Better Work Your Brain

The reactive and creative qualities of both leadership performance and resiliency relate to patterns of activity in specific networks and regions in the brain that we all have.

Chapter 2, page 38

You can consciously build a more resilient brain to live a more creative and meaningful life.

Chapter 2, page 71

Now that chapter 1 has set the first foundational layer of the science of Conscious Leadership, chapter 2 explores your biology that enables it.

Most of us would say we experience both reactive, low-performance leadership qualities, *and* creative, high-performance leadership qualities—sometimes shifting between the two multiple times a day! Why? *It's how our brain naturally functions!* Chapter 2 provides a user's guide for the brain specifically tailored for leaders, so you can better understand how your brain works to optimize your energy and performance. In doing so, you'll discover how to make the shift from reactivity to creativity whenever you need it, and leverage the best your brain has to offer.

In sharing this brief overview of how your brain works, my hope is that you'll realize there's nothing wrong with you when you feel stressed. Your brain's stress response to a perceived threat is simply a result of how your brain is programmed—not just from childhood, but from millennia of evolutionary history. We are hardwired to fight or take flight to protect ourselves from threat and harm. This response isn't bad or wrong—it's adaptive, especially in the face of short-term stressors, like being chased by a predator.

Today, our brains still operate very similarly to the way they did in prehistoric times, but we now have different types of stressors that are more prolonged, such as worrying about our finances or difficult people in our lives, where our fight-or-flight threat responses over the long term can do more harm than good. The good news is that we now also have the science to better understand the brain and manage modern stress. We now know there are other types of stress responses that are far more helpful than fight-or-flight when dealing with these prolonged stressors. So if your brain is your prehistoric-age operating system, these neuroscientific discoveries are your new software updates that will help you not only handle greater levels of stress but actually leverage even more adaptive stress responses to help you sustain higher levels of performance.

In chapter 2, you learn why your brain feels scrambled when you get overwhelmed by stress, and why an ongoing threat response predisposes you to burnout. You'll also learn which part of your brain best serves as its CEO in order to maximize your brain's ability to manage and leverage stress, allowing you to proactively shift between reactivity and creativity and transform burnout into resiliency. (As a bonus, you'll also discover how you can avoid stepping on a stress-laden landmine when you get home from work.) Finally, you'll discover the difference between your brain and your mind—and how a particular state of mind—conscious awareness—allows you to proactively shift between the states of reactivity and creativity.

Key Points

- We all experience states of reactivity and creativity because they relate to patterns of brain activity we all have. In short, the state of *reactivity* results when we feel threatened and our lower survival-oriented parts of our brain take control, and the state of *creativity* results when our higher, more cognitively flexible parts of our brain are in control.

- One helpful way to think about our brain's organizational structure is the concept of the **triune brain**. According to this concept, first developed by Dr. Paul MacLean in the 1960s, our brain developed evolutionarily from the bottom up and from the back forward and has three main parts:

the reptilian brain (brain stem and basal ganglia), the mammalian brain (limbic system), and the neocortex (which includes the prefrontal cortex).

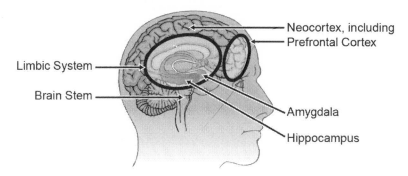

> Your **brain stem** is involved in crucial survival needs including controlling your respiration, blood pressure, and heart rate as well as your fight and flight responses. Your **basal ganglia** are involved in movement, habit formation, reward, and motivation.

> Your **limbic system** is responsible for your primal drives related to feeding, sex, and bonding in intimate relationships. Most notably, it also plays a key role in your memory and emotions. One key part of the limbic system is the **amygdala**, which stores emotional memories and helps keep you safe. It's predisposed to look for problems or danger rather than savoring joyful moments. If a person or event matches for threat, the amygdala sends signals directly to your brain stem and your hypothalamus to mobilize your fight-or-flight responses throughout your body so you can fend off your attacker or get away now.

Together, the brain stem/basal ganglia and the limbic system are primitive, subcortical, subconscious structures critical to your basic survival needs, moving you toward immediate pleasure and away from pain. While these subconscious regions of the brain developed to protect us from physical harm, they may also be responsible for some of the low-performance leadership qualities we described earlier, such as becoming highly controlling, protective, or overly compliant.

> The third part of your triune brain, the **neocortex**, is vital to your conscious awareness and engaging high-performance, Conscious

Leadership. It includes your ability to strategize, make good decisions, achieve your desired results, connect well with others, and maintain self-awareness and self-composure in times of stress.

- The concept of the triune brain maps beautifully to **Maslow's Hierarchy of Needs,** simplified here with three layers that build upon the other. The needs of **safety**, **love and belonging**, and **significance** generally correspond with the brain stem, the limbic system, and the neocortex.

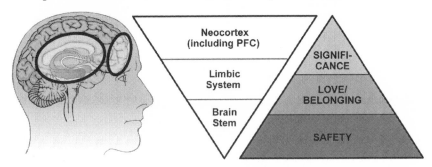

Once your lower Maslowian needs are met, you're able to address the next level of needs with its corresponding region of the brain. For example, when you feel safe, you can more fully engage your capacity for empathy, love, and compassion. And when your sense of love and belonging is secure, you can think more creatively, which puts yourself in a position to actualize your full potential and experience greater meaning and significance in your life.

- On the flip side, when you're unable to meet your Maslowian needs for a prolonged period of time, you tend to experience **burnout**. In fact, the three characteristics of burnout also correspond with Maslow's hierarchy.

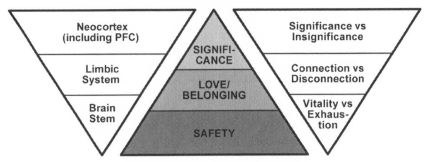

If you're not having your physiological and safety needs met, you are continually drawing upon resources from the survival-oriented parts of your brain—which can leave you in a state of **exhaustion**. And as you pour resources into your safety and survival circuits, you forego meeting your love and belonging needs and can experience a sense of **disconnection**. Finally, as you simultaneously withdraw your resources away from the circuits in the cortex and PFC that enable you to experience self-esteem and self-actualization, you can be left with a reduced sense of personal accomplishment, or feeling of **insignificance**.

- On the other hand, meeting your hierarchy of needs results in resiliency against burnout. For example, when you are able to meet your physiological and safety needs, you can experience a sense of **vitality**. When you meet your love and belonging needs, you can experience a sense of **connection**. And when you meet your needs for self-esteem and are able to self-actualize, you can experience a great sense of accomplishment and **significance** in your life.

- The three parts of our triune brain are not separate but are highly networked. What directs this highly networked activity is known as your *mind*.

- Although there are differing views, one compelling definition of the mind comes from Dr. Dan Siegel and his colleagues: "the mind is an embodied and relational process that regulates the flow of energy and information within the brain and between brains."

- In particular, two main streams of mental activity influence whether you move toward reactivity or creativity: **the threat of stress and self-doubt**, and **inspiration**.

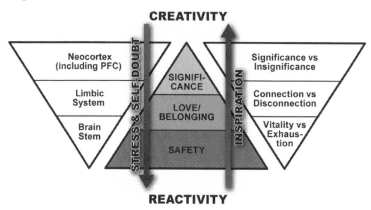

- A number of researchers point out that we feel threatened when the **demands** we experience exceed the **resources** we have to handle them.

- Stress and self-doubt are commonly thought of as two distinct but related experiences. **Stress** asks the question, "Can I handle it?" **Self-doubt** can be a subset of this kind of stress, where we further ask, "And how will I value myself in the process of handling this stressful situation?" According to these definitions, when we feel stress or self-doubt we may feel disempowered, feeling we can't handle things or that we are not good enough. Thus stress and self-doubt themselves can intensify the demands on us, deplete our resources, and make us feel threatened.

- Whenever your perceived demands exceed your perceived resources, and you feel unsafe as you experience stress or self-doubt, your threat response is triggered, activating a specific type of **sympathetic nervous system** reaction that revs you up and drives your flow of mental activity into your survival circuits and creates a state of reactivity.

  When you experience intense stress, it can result in "amygdala highjack," when your PFC can get taken offline from a perceived threat.

- Remember that reactivity is not always "bad." It can have many adaptive advantages, especially keeping you safe in short-term situations. The key is to determine whether reactivity is doing more harm than good in a certain situation.

- Just as the threat of stress and self-doubt leads to reactivity, the experience of inspiration leads to creativity. Changing your **mindset** about stress and self-doubt—viewing it as an asset rather than solely a threat—can fuel the stream of inspiration and therefore the state of creativity.

- Kelly McGonigal, a health psychologist at Stanford, offers a broader and more empowering and transformative definition of stress that facilitates the shift from reactivity to creativity: "Stress is what arises when something you care about is at stake." This definition implies that stress (or self-doubt) is there to help you. Hence, it enhances your inner resources rather than depletes them. This shift in mindset may convert your threat reactions into even more adaptive stress responses.

- In addition to your **threat response** to stress and self-doubt, there are at least two other responses where your resources are sufficient to meet your demands, both of which may facilitate creativity:

  > The **challenge response** enables you to leverage all of your inner resources, including your knowledge, skills, and the energy of stress itself, to effectively meet the challenges you face.

  > The **tend-and-befriend response** enables you to mobilize your external resources of social support as well as collaborate in difficult situations.

- These three stress responses also map to Maslow's Hierarchy of Needs. The threat response, which corresponds to safety, drives your mental stream into a state of reactivity. Conversely, the tend-and-befriend response, which corresponds with love and belonging, and the challenge response, which corresponds with significance, both drive your mental stream up your hierarchy of needs into states of creativity (see figure above on page 19 of this summary).

- As you move up Maslow's hierarchy, you will notice that your creativity engages your higher cortical circuits, including your PFC. However, it's also important to point our that these higher levels of your brain integrate all levels below it. Because your brain is highly networked, creativity is not just a function of your PFC but is indeed a **whole-brain process**— although in many ways it is orchestrated by your PFC that plays a key role in integrating all layers of the brain.

- The state of creativity may also include both **divergent thinking** (to create novel ideas) and **convergent thinking** (to refine those novel ideas into useful ideas).

- It also includes moments of **peak performance**—a "Maslow moment" of self-actualization, or what Mihaly Csikszentmihalyi calls "flow."

- Each of us has the capacity for reactivity and creativity at any moment. We tend to flip-flop back and forth between these states in a dynamic **reactivity-creativity equilibrium**. Again, the two factors that impact the amount of time you tend to spend in reactivity versus creativity are stress and self-doubt (when experienced as threats), and inspiration.

- To lead well from within, you need to ensure you have the best driver in the driver's seat to meet life's demands. Research shows that you can regulate the activity in your subconscious limbic system with your PFC to rapidly recover from stress and reactivity and cultivate a more creative mindset and greater resiliency.

- Research also show that the brain is moldable, or "plastic." It continually rewires and reshapes itself, even growing new neurons throughout your lifespan, in a process called *neuroplasticity*. And what's profoundly encouraging is that you have the power to rewire your own brain through your thoughts, experiences, and habitual practices in what has been called "*self-directed neuroplasticity.*"

- Therefore, you can not only learn how to better work your brain, but you can create a better one, too. What it takes is **conscious awareness and your ability to focus your attention on what matters most**. This brings us to the third layer of our foundation for Conscious Leadership, which focuses on the practice of **mindfulness.**

How to Better Work Your Brain with Mindfulness

To successfully navigate back to high-performance leadership, you need to both more consciously work your brain to enhance your internal resources and develop your resilience to stay on the path of high performance, especially when external and internal demands of stress, uncertainty, or self-doubt threaten to derail you. The solution is mindfulness.

Chapter 3, page 73

As chapter 2 explained, our mind plays a key role in directing the flow of energy and information within our brain. The practice of mindfulness helps you engage and direct the focus of your attention with conscious awareness, a state of mind involving your higher cortical circuits and PFC that allows you to shift between reactivity and creativity when it would better serve.

According to Jon Kabat-Zinn, who inspired much of the research and popularized mindfulness in the West as a secular practice, "mindfulness means paying attention in a particular way; on purpose, in the present moment, and nonjudgmentally." It enables you to be more aware and present, less prone to being swept away by pain and distraction, and more purposeful in focusing your energy and attention on what is truly most meaningful in your life.

In this chapter, you'll learn more about what mindfulness is, its history, its proven benefits, and how to experience its benefits starting now. Rather than overidentifying with, being swept away by, or judging yourself for any particular reactive thoughts or feelings (like anger, fear, or resentment), you'll learn how to observe your thoughts and feelings with openness, curiosity, and kindness. This allows you to experience a greater sense of clarity, presence, and equanimity that characterizes Conscious Leadership.

Key Points

- Various forms of mindfulness have been practiced for thousands of years in many of the wisdom traditions, including Hinduism, Daoism, Buddhism, Christianity, Islam, and Judaism.

- In 1979, Jon Kabat-Zinn began teaching mindfulness as a way to help patients deal with their suffering from pain and chronic illness when it could not be fully managed by the healthcare system. His evidence-based, nonreligious Mindfulness-Based Stress Reduction Program has been taught at over seven hundred hospitals worldwide. Its mindfulness practices have inspired those shared in *Leading Well from Within.*

- In addition to healthcare, mindfulness is now being practiced profitably in virtually every setting, including in the military, the legal system, law enforcement, government, and business.

- A large body of research supports the benefits of mindfulness. Repeated studies have shown that mindfulness reduces anxiety, depression, pain, stress, and distress. It's been shown to benefit a wide variety of conditions such as ADHD, eating disorders, addictions, irritable bowel syndrome, psoriasis, and other health concerns. And it's been shown to increase our internal quality of life and productivity at work (and thus businesses' profitability).

- Further neuroscientific research has shown that mindfulness can help you reshape your brain to manage stress better, transform your stress response from threat to challenge, shift from a reactive to a creative mindset, and live a healthier, more engaged, more joyful, and more productive life.

- To unpack the phrase in Jon Kabat-Zinn's definition, "Mindfulness means paying attention in a particular way; on purpose, in the present moment, and nonjudgmentally":

  - "On purpose" refers to being aware of your intention in practicing mindfulness, or your "why" for practicing it.

  - "Paying attention" refers to the way you learn to direct and redirect your focus of attention on the contents of your consciousness, moment by moment, in the present. (And what you pay attention to grows.)

> ➤ "In a particular way" refers to the attitude or qualities you bring to your practice. While a cold, analytical, or judgmental lens can create a hard-driving or self-critical way of being, the nonjudgmental qualities of **openness**, **curiosity**, and **kindness** promote a sense of equanimity and ease.

- In a further resonance with Maslow's Hierarchy of Needs and your adaptive stress responses, kindness facilitates your tend-and-befriend response to meet your love and belonging needs and, and curiosity engages your challenge response and growth mindset to meet your needs for self-actualization and significance.

- In Japanese kanji, mindfulness (*nen*) is represented by a character that combines the elements of "heart" and "mind," nestled under a "roof" representing "now." This character captures the very essence of mindfulness—bringing conscious awareness with your heart and mind to your moment of now.

- In this chapter, I invite you to experience a brief mindfulness practice where you focus your attention on your breathing (see pages 83–86, or **Mindfulness Practice: Focusing on Your Breathing**, available as a bonus at SuperSmartHealth.com/Book). We then reflect together on your experience of this practice and the application of mindfulness to high-performance Conscious Leadership.

- In simplest terms, mindfulness is the power to *notice* and *choose*. Your mind's ability to notice and choose engages your PFC, the CEO of your brain. And at your hub of awareness, with your mind engaging the CEO of your brain, you are truly centered and have tremendous power to marshal your inner resources to meet any demand and lead well from within.

- To cultivate your practice of mindfulness, you can practice focusing on your breathing for at least five to fifteen minutes, twice a day, as well as more informally integrate mindfulness throughout your day by bringing mindful awareness to whatever you are doing at least for a few moments each hour, starting now.

CHAPTER 4

Introducing the 4 in 4 Framework to Engage Conscious Leadership

The 4 in 4 Framework to Engage Conscious Leadership provides you with science-backed skills and mindfulness-based practices to become more aware and shift from the state of reactivity to creativity in the heat of the moment, as well as rewire your brain to shift your equilibrium so that you may also become less reactive and more creative over time.

Chapter 4, page 100

While mindfulness provides a powerful foundation for the Conscious Leader, you can still be pulled off track by stress and self-doubt or not be fully clear on your purpose that gives your life a sense of direction. In this chapter, we'll build upon the foundations of the research supporting Conscious Leadership, brain science, and mindfulness by introducing a *framework* that includes the skills and practices to help you navigate stress and stay on track with what's truly meaningful in your life: **The 4 in 4 Framework to Engage Conscious Leadership.**

According to most of my clients, their obstacles to achieving peak performance tend to fall into two categories: they're either overwhelmed with the threat of stress or self-doubt, or they're lacking the focus, vision, or inspiration that energizes them to do their best work. The 4 in 4 Framework is a system that enables you to effectively navigate and leverage your stress and self-doubt so you can focus your attention on what matters most to you. It allows you to clarify an inspirational life vision and create strategies to optimize your health, your relationships, and your productivity. Even better, it will help you cultivate resiliency to burnout in high-stress environments and even expand your capacity for peak performance!

27

Key Points

- Many people think that the relationship between stress and performance is linear—that is, you perform at your best when your stress is lowest, and your performance decreases as your stress level increases. But stress levels that are too high *or* too low can cause your performance to suffer. Psychologists Robert Yerkes and John Dodson discovered this relationship between stress (arousal) and performance in the early 1900s, as represented by the bell-shaped curve shown below.

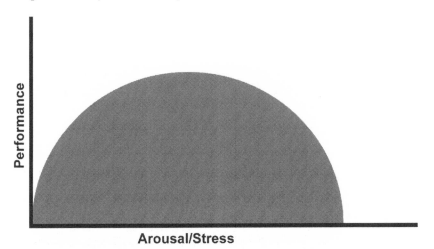

Arousal/Stress

- Therefore, learning skills within the two domains of resiliency—the ability to recover from the distress of stress *and* to leverage a healthy level of stress to lean in to meaningful challenges—is the key to optimizing your energy and navigating toward the peak of your performance curve.

  Steps 1 and 2 of the 4 in 4 Framework help you address the first domain, allowing you to climb up the right side of the performance curve when stress and self-doubt are too high. Steps 3 and 4 can help you address the second domain, allowing you climb up the left side of the performance curve when positive stress energy and inspiration is low.

- These steps also help expand your inner resources to meet your Maslowian Hierarchy of Needs. Steps 1 and 2 help you establish your safety and love/belonging needs as you learn to shift from a threat response to a challenge or tend-and-befriend response. Steps 3 and 4 help you further meet your love/belonging needs and your need for significance.

- The 4 in 4 Framework is so named because it has four steps with four parts to each step.

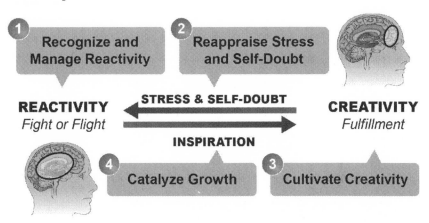

> **Step 1: Recognizing and Managing Reactivity** helps you identify when you feel threatened by stress and self-doubt and take the edge off your reactions. It helps you feel more in control and allows you to respond more wisely with a powerful and simple skill that has been scientifically proven to calm your reactive response within seconds. It also includes a mindfulness practice to help you rewire your brain to turn this skill into a more helpful habit.

> In **Step 2: Appraising and Reappraising Stress and Self-Doubt,** you'll explore how you can shift your mindset about stress and self-doubt, as well as neutralize their underlying triggers that may well have their hooks in you. The skill and mindfulness practice of Step 2 allow you to reappraise both your personal triggers and your mindset about stress and self-doubt. As a result, you feel more secure and confident even when facing the most challenging circumstances.

> **Step 3: Cultivating Creativity** teaches you how to identify your core values and strengths, guided by a list of factors that overlap with the keys to what Positive Psychology founder Martin Seligman calls a "flourishing" life. You then incorporate your specific values and strengths into a step-by-step process that helps you further clarify

your life vision, implement strategies, and manifest specific and measurable results in your health, relationships, and productivity. Step 3 also teaches you mindfulness practices to enhance your wellness and vitality, connect more deeply with yourself and others, and become more creative and impactful while serving at home and at work.

> **Step 4: Catalyzing Growth** provides you with a life-changing skill that engages your deepest source of inspiration so you can stay aligned moment by moment with what's truly important in your life, especially when stress and self-doubt threaten to derail you. As you learn to ask better questions mindfully, find better answers, make wiser decisions, and take action that's more aligned with your core values and vision for your flourishing life, you create a more inspired internal dialogue, which enables you to better tap into your inner resources over time. In many ways, because Step 4 catalyzes the first three steps and your ongoing growth, it may be the most important step of all.

• Finally, using the power of neuroplasticity, the 4 in 4 Framework doesn't just help you achieve your peak performance, as shown in the figure below—it can actually expand it!

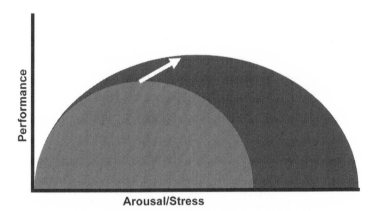

Part 2

Applying the 4 in 4 Framework
to Lead Well from Within

Step 1: Recognizing and Managing Reactivity

The benefit of doing the spadework to recognize your patterns of reactivity is that you can take the edge off your reactive responses earlier, right when they occur. Instead of your reactivity leading you to say or do things you may regret, becoming more aware and recognizing your reactivity enables you to lead well from within, so you can modify your behavior before you overstep your bounds and do harm to yourself or others.

Chapter 5, page 114

When we experience the discomfort of stress and self-doubt, we often want to do whatever it takes to get rid of it—right now! But the first step to shifting from a reactive to a creative mindset is not to instantly shut reactivity down, but to mindfully notice it with openness, curiosity, and kindness. Reactivity can also be an adaptive response, and it's always an important teacher. The key question is whether your reactivity is doing more harm than good in the moment. If it is, you can then take steps to manage it, so it doesn't overwhelm you. Instead, it can become positive energy for your best response. That's exactly what Step 1 helps you do.

I begin the chapter by sharing how I unexpectedly found myself on the edge of a panic attack during a key presentation. The story illustrates how Step 1 saved me from disaster in a high-stakes situation. In chapter 5, I'll show you how to do the same. You'll learn how to identify the different types of stress responses (the threat response, the challenge response, and the tend-and-befriend response); how to recognize your own reactive sensations, thoughts, feelings, and behaviors in the moment; and the four steps to manage your reactivity when you find it's doing more harm than good. You'll also learn a mindfulness technique to strengthen your capacity to practice Step 1 in the heat of the moment.

Key Points

- When your threat response to stress is activated, and you're unaware of it, you can get lost in a spiral of reactivity—a dynamic interplay between your **physical sensations, thoughts, emotions and feelings,** and **behaviors.**

  > Your reactive **sensations** represent your body moving from a physiological state of "rest and digest" to one of "fight or flight." You experience the same physical responses to perceived threats whether they're physical or psychological, such as the shutting down of your digestive system, your heart racing, hyper-focusing or scrambled thinking, and others.

  > Your reactive **thoughts** tend to fall into four categories: all the bad things that could happen, the regrets of your past, what's wrong with you, and what's wrong with others.

  > **Emotions** occur when a stimulus triggers a complex psychological state that includes a physiological response, interpretations of the event, facial and vocal expressions, and a behavioral response. **Feelings** are your subjective experience of your emotions. Reactive emotions may include irritation, frustration, anger, and hostility when energy is high, and sadness, depression, shame, and hopelessness when energy is low.

  > Reactive **behaviors** often fall into the descriptive categories we used for low-performance leadership: in the controlling dimension, it can include the "fight" for control, for power, or to prove self-worth. In the complying dimension, it can include pleasing others to gain validation and self-worth, following rules rigidly, or being passive and indecisive. In the protecting dimension, it can include "flight" away from others by acting inaccessible, aloof, emotionally distant, and uncaring; or the "fight" to prove self-worth through arrogance, intellectual domination, and being highly judgmental.

- This interconnected spiral of reactive sensations, thoughts, feelings, and behaviors can be highly adaptive if you're truly in danger in the moment. However, it can also cause you to overreact out of proportion and cause more harm than good—causing you to fall further down the right side of the stress and performance curve.

- So once you recognize your reactive responses, the key question is, *In this moment, is my reactivity likely to do me and others more harm than good?* If it is, you can use these **four steps to manage your reactivity** (see pages 128–132).

  ➤ Step 1 is to simply **pause**, allowing yourself to mindfully be with whatever sensations, thoughts, and feelings you are experiencing. As best you can, release any resistance and relax into whatever you are experiencing with a sense of openness, curiosity, and kindness.

  ➤ Step 2 is to **take three heart-centered, soft-belly breaths** to help activate your parasympathetic nervous system (PNS), the "brake" that regulates your revved-up sympathetic drive.

  ➤ Step 3 is to **"name it to tame it,"** to quote Dan Siegel. Naming your emotions mindfully has been shown to further activate your PFC and soothe your revved-up amygdala that's driving your reactivity.

  ➤ Step 4 is to **consider your best response**. Now that you've activated your PFC and have taken the edge off your reactivity, you can think more clearly about how to best respond next. First, make sure you've taken care of your physical and safety needs. Then ask yourself what you want most in this situation, and how you might best act to achieve this outcome. If you still find yourself reactive, move on to Step 2 in the 4 in 4 Framework, which will help you learn from and work through the underlying issues that are continuing to drive your reactive response.

- The mindfulness practice to accompany your new skills of recognizing and managing your reactivity is the formal practice of **Naming Your Experiences.** It helps strengthen your capacity to take the edge off your reactivity in the heat of the moment and prepare you to more easily call upon this skill in difficult situations when you need it the most. See pages 132–135 for full instructions, or SuperSmartHealth.com/Book.

CHAPTER 6

Step 2: Reappraising Stress and Self-Doubt

If you approach stress [and self-doubt] as an asset, you can find the good in what it has to offer. You can learn, grow, and become even stronger and more resilient. You can leverage that stress into energy to fuel your transformation and a more meaningful life.

Chapter 6, page 139

Step 2 moves beyond simply recognizing and taking the edge off your reactivity to uncover the underlying stress and self-doubt that is driving your reactive responses to begin with.

I begin the chapter with the story of one of my clients, "Chris," whose own reactive behaviors (including drinking one or two bottles of wine a night) were causing him even greater stress and self-doubt, further increasing those reactive behaviors, and making things even worse. For this deeper work of reappraising stress and self-doubt, and as Chris discovered in our work together, before addressing your triggers of stress and self-doubt, it's helpful to first address your *mindset* about stress and self-doubt. Once you defuse your "stress about being stressed," often the triggers themselves become much more manageable.

In this chapter, you'll learn first how to change your own relationship with stress and self-doubt so you can view them as potential assets to help you move through life's challenges. Then you'll discover how to both appraise (evaluate) and reappraise (reframe) the underlying triggers that are causing them in the first place.

Key Points

- The first part of Step 2 is to **reappraise your mindset about stress and self-doubt**. Transforming stress and self-doubt into an asset can improve your health, productivity, and physiology—perhaps more than if you hadn't experienced them at all!

  - ➤ You can **reappraise your stress mindset** by understanding how it indeed can be an asset, helping you to mobilize energy and resources to take care of whatever is most at stake for you. Further, by approaching your stress mindfully—with openness, curiosity, and kindness—you can shift your threat response to a challenge or a tend-and-befriend response, whichever is more helpful in the given situation.

  - ➤ To help illustrate how to **reappraise your self-doubt mindset**, I share my story about learning to transform my own experience with self-doubt in medical school, and helping my fellow students to do the same. I then share the research I conducted on self-doubt at San Francisco International Airport, showing how self-doubt is normal and even useful. Here mindfulness is also the key. By simply observing your thoughts and feelings of self-doubt with openness, curiosity, and kindness, you can reflect on and even be thankful for what self-doubt has to teach you.

- Reappraising your stress and self-doubt mindset now makes the second part of Step 2, **Appraising and Reappraising Your Triggers of Stress and Self-Doubt**, even easier.

  - ➤ **Triggers of stress** can be both physical and psychological. David Rock, Director of the NeuroLeadership Institute, identifies some of the most common psychological stressors with the mnemonic SCARF: threats to Status, Certainty, Autonomy, Relatedness, and Fairness.

  - ➤ Common **triggers to self-doubt** are judgment and criticism, rejection and abandonment, neglect and abuse, failure to live up to standards and expectations, losing things that make you feel worthy, and transition.

  - ➤ Although we often think of triggers of stress and self-doubt as external events, usually it's your *beliefs* or *perceptions* about these external events that are your true triggers.

- **The Appraise-Reappraise Method** helps you reframe painful perceptions with two questions to help you *appraise* your current perceptions of stress and self-doubt and two questions to help you *reappraise* them (see pages 157–164).

  - > Question 1 is simply, **"What happened?"** Here you clearly distinguish between facts and perceptions by establishing "just the facts" about what happened.

  - > Question 2 is **"What are my *beliefs* about what happened?"** Here you have the opportunity to identify your beliefs about the facts or events, and note how very often your negative beliefs about facts adds to your suffering. Your deepest fears often lie in a cascading set of beliefs—a "fear tree" that you can map by sequentially asking, "If this fear were true, what would happen next?" When you can go no further, you may discover what lies at the root of your stress or self-doubt: your deepest fear. Once you have distinguished the facts from your beliefs and have done the spadework of identifying the root fear beneath your beliefs, you can move on to the next two questions and reappraise your beliefs to transform your pain and open new possibilities for moving forward.

  - > Question 3 is **"Am I certain my belief is really true?"** Much of what we believe is distorted thinking or even pure fabrication. So ask yourself, "Is how I'm seeing this really true?" Or, "What is the evidence that this should be so?" If you can shake up your limiting beliefs, you can make room for new growth in your life and open the door to viewing your triggers in more helpful ways.

  - > Question 4 is **"How can I view this situation differently?"** Here you consider how you can see things in a new way that either brings you less stress or self-doubt, or better yet, leverages your stress or self-doubt to achieve the outcomes that matter most to you.

- Research shows that mindfulness can powerfully facilitate reappraisal. Functional MRI scans of the brain show that reappraisal activates your PFC and deactivates your limbic system, and it's most pronounced in individuals who score high on tests of mindfulness. Mindfulness allows you to pause, think, and respond more clearly, rather than reacting to difficult situations subconsciously from your emotional, fear-based brain.

- To take advantage of the benefits of mindfulness, you can also engage the practice of **Working the Appraise-Reappraise Method Mindfully**. For step-by-step instructions, visit SuperSmartHealth.com/Book.

- Another formal mindfulness practice that can help you more effectively establish Step 2 as a habit in your life is the formal practice of **Loving-Kindness**. It rewires your brain with a circuit of unconditional self-acceptance and a deep knowing that you love and accept yourself no matter what, self-doubt and all. This practice helps to meet your Maslowian needs for safety and love and belonging. For step-by-step instructions, see "part one" of this practice on pages 166–169 or at SuperSmartHealth.com/Book.

CHAPTER 7

Cultivating Creativity

Now that you've learned how to defuse your reactivity, in Step 3 you'll be making the turn into creativity, where you'll feel inspired to optimize your health, relationships, and overall productivity. Here you will create an ideal life vision where you will clarify and manifest what matters most to you. Instead of running fear-based simulations about all that could go wrong, you'll be running success-based simulations to create the life you want to live—where you feel more energized, fulfilled, and resilient.

Chapter 7, page 171

In Steps 1 and 2 of the 4 in 4 Framework, with your new skills of managing your reactivity and reappraising your stress and self-doubt, you have learned to cultivate a deeper sense of safety and confidence within. Now that you have liberated significant energy from the base of your hierarchy of needs, you can make the shift from safety towards your love, belonging, and mattering needs to cultivate creativity and experience a whole new world of possibility and growth.

In Step 3, you'll learn a powerful step-by-step process to leverage this energy to focus on what is truly important in your life—optimizing your health and vitality, deepening your most important relationships, and meeting your highest needs to find greater success and significance in your life at work and at home.

Key Points

- In this chapter, the **VSIR Process** teaches you how to optimize your health, relationships, and productivity, or any other area of your life that's important to you.

- VSIR stands for **vision**, **strategy**, **implementation**, and **results**, as shown in the figure below.

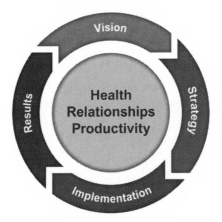

> Your **vision** is an image of your ideal future. It encapsulates your purpose and passion for being and generates the guiding force of inspiration in your life. This part of the VSIR cycle answers the question, "What is my vision for a meaningful life?" (See pages 175–183.)

> Your **strategies** are the key components (i.e., headings and subheadings) of your plan to achieve your vision. For example, if a specific aspect of your vision is a mental picture of you thriving with health and vitality, your strategy may be to consider how to *take out the bad stuff* in your life, like toxic health habits, and put in the good stuff, like *eating well*, *exercising*, getting refreshing *sleep*, and practicing *mindfulness*. You could also identify sub-strategies. For example, under *eating well*, you may find it helpful to subscribe to what author Michael Pollan suggests, "Eat [real] food, not too much, mostly plants." (See pages 187–203.)

➤ **Implementation** refers to the specific steps you're taking to execute your plan. Once you've come up with your strategies for a certain area, then write down exactly what you're going to do to put that strategy into action today, tomorrow, next week, etc. For example, to implement your health strategy of eating well, you might create a to-do list that includes when you will dispose of all unhealthy foods in your pantry, your healthy-eating grocery list, and when and where you will shop. Then you put that plan into action. (See pages 187–203.)

➤ Your **results** serve as stepping stones you can follow toward manifesting your vision. To be pragmatic and effective, ensure your results are SMART: Specific, Measurable, Aligned to your vision, Realistic, and Time-framed.

When you begin the VSIR Process, after clarifying your vision, it can be most helpful "to look left before you look right," first moving counterclockwise from your vision to clarify your intended results for your health, relationships, and productivity. Then you move clockwise through strategic implementation and again to results, where you reflect on whether you have achieved your results in each of these areas. (See pages 183–187 and 203–204.)

• The VSIR Process is an iterative process. If, after taking action, you find you are not meeting your specific results in your intended time frame, you can reiterate the cycle by reflecting on ways you may want to refine your vision, strategies, or implementation process, or consider whether your results were realistic. Then take action to run the cycle again and again.

• Just as you can work the Appraise-Reappraise Method in Step 2 as a mindfulness practice, you can also engage in **Working the VSIR Process Mindfully** to either initiate or refine whatever work you've already done. For step-by-step instructions for this practice, visit SuperSmartHealth.com/Book.

• Another mindfulness practice to enhance your practice of Step 3 is the **Energy Optimizing Body Scan**, an adaptation of Jon Kabat-Zinn's Body Scan. This practice enables you to more fully appreciate and connect with the experience of being in your body and its abundance of energy, which may give you a deep sense of vitality. As you do, you may find yourself more inclined and motivated to more fully care for your body, to nourish it with positive health habits and extend yourself (and others) a greater measure of tenderness, kindness, and compassion. For step-by-step instructions, visit SuperSmartHealth.com/Book.

- Yet another helpful mindfulness practice is one of **Mindfully Engaging Your Energy within Your Hierarchy of Needs**. This practice also builds on the Energy Optimizing Body Scan above to help you feel more energized, loving, and connected to purpose and significance in your life. For step-by-step instructions, see pages 207–209, or visit SuperSmartHealth.com/Book.

CHAPTER 8

Step 4: Catalyzing Growth

Step 4 helps you catalyze your growth from the first three steps by transforming your internal dialogue, so you can continually make the turn from reactivity to creativity and stay aligned, moment by moment, with your flow of inspiration and what's truly most important in your life.

Chapter 8, page 212

Even with all the skills and practices you've learned in Steps 1, 2, and 3, ongoing stress and self-doubt can trigger reactivity at any moment and throw you off track. Also, your internal dialogue can create an undertow that keeps you susceptible to your threat response and ongoing reactivity, which may limit your ability to attain and sustain the vision of your life well lived. Step 4 teaches you a four-step process to engage in a more inspired internal dialogue, which enables you to more fully tap into your internal resources for creating your meaningful life.

To begin this chapter, I share the story of how I discovered the power of Step 4 unexpectedly through my work as an expert in evidence-based medicine (EBM), the gold standard by which all healthcare decisions are now made. Ironically, I had become intensely disoriented about the direction of my career in EBM, and the question that kept coming to me was "What's wrong with me?"—which triggered an overwhelming threat response and left me locked down in a painful contortion of despair. Then something miraculous happened: a different question occurred to me. I found myself asking, "How can I find my way home?"

In an instant, my entire outlook and physiology changed. In my amazement, I recognized that all I did was *ask a better question!* That's when I realized the circular, four-step EBM process of (1) **asking** the right clinical questions, (2) **finding** the best available scientific research to answer these questions, (3) **evaluating** the research, and (4) **applying** the research to make the best possible healthcare decisions had given me the foundation for helping myself as well as others find their way home. I adapted this process to result in what has now become Step 4 of the 4 in 4 Framework.

With Step 4, you will discover how to catalyze your growth and expand your capacity for peak performance in all areas of your life through the simple miracle of asking better questions. Although it's a simple step, it may be the most powerful step of all.

Key Points

- An adaptation of the four-step EBM framework, Step 4 is a circular, four-step process that enables you to (1) **ask** better questions, (2) **find** more inspiring answers, (3) **evaluate** your answers to ensure they feel right, and (4) **apply** your answers by taking purposeful action in your life.

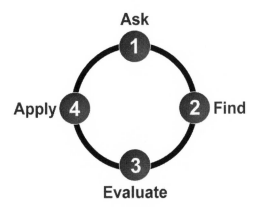

- The questions you **ask** set the direction of your life. Whether you frame your questions creatively or reactively makes all the difference in whether you more deeply establish your growth mindset and become a creative person, or you close the doorway to opportunity and growth. Steps 1, 2, and 3 include some of the key questions that help catalyze your growth in making the shift from reactivity to creativity. (See pages 215–219.)

> To **find** the answers to your questions, you can search either externally from trusted resources, or internally. This step focuses on the latter approach, creating optimal brain conditions so your answers can find *you*. A variety of practices can help you optimize your mental state to find more insightful answers to your questions. (See pages 220–223.)

> To **evaluate** your answers, you reflect on whether the answers you receive are aligned with your deepest values—whether they feel right—or are more about simply wanting to feel relieved or feel good. (See pages 223–224.)

> Next, you **apply** your answers by taking purposeful action on them, summoning the courage and gathering the support you need to follow through. (See pages 224–226.)

> After you take action to apply your answers, you complete the cycle by returning to the first step in Step 4 to **ask** your next question: "Is what I'm doing working?" If not, you ask more questions. If so, consider it an invitation to experience awe and appreciation for whatever you credit as the source of your inspiration for guiding this process. (See pages 227–228.)

- **Step 4 is itself a mindfulness practice you can use in your everyday life.** Typically, it's preceded by an "invitation" or a "call," where you may be experiencing "limbic" reactivity (Step 1), discomfort due to underlying triggers of stress or self-doubt (Step 2), or a restlessness or desire to close the gap between your life now and your life well lived (Step 3). When these invitations come, approach them with a sense of openness, curiosity, and kindness, and then mindfully move through each of the four steps of Step 4. For step-by-step instructions, see pages 228–230 or visit SuperSmartHealth.com/Book.

Part 3

Applying the 4 in 4 Framework
to Lead Well in the World

Cycles of Reactivity and Creativity

Since we are wired to connect, we don't just experience reactivity and creativity personally, but in cycles of reactivity and creativity with others as well.

Chapter 9, page 252

In part 2 of *Leading Well from Within*, you learned how to apply the four steps of the 4 in 4 Framework to recognize and manage your reactivity, reappraise your stress and self-doubt, leverage this energy to cultivate creativity around what matters most in your life, and further catalyze your growth with a powerful process of mindfulness-based inquiry. Now that you have the knowledge, skills, and practices to lead well from within, you're ready for part 3, where you will learn to apply this framework to lead well in the world.

Chapter 9 begins with the brain science of connection, where you will more deeply understand how the systems that facilitate social connection drive the human experience, why it's so devastating to feel rejection (and rewarding to feel connected), and how we regulate the emotions and impulses that can impair our social functioning. You'll discover that just as individuals oscillate between states of reactivity and creativity, groups and cultures also experience similar cycles of creativity and cycles of reactivity. Then, in the next chapter, you'll learn how to apply the 4 in 4 Framework to resolve conflicts and nurture your most important relationships.

Key Points

- Your brain is wired to socially connect through multiple neural systems and networks, including social pain and reward, mirror neurons, emotional and cognitive empathy, PFC regulation, and key components of your autonomic nervous system.

- Research shows that the activity of these networks manifests not just in your internal experience, but in your facial expressions and the tone of your voice. Altogether these systems and networks mean you don't experience reactivity and creativity in isolation. As a species, we are intimately linked with each other in ways that are socially contagious.

- In other words, your reactivity or creativity is usually obvious to others, and they respond accordingly, triggering **cycles of reactivity and creativity** within relationships.

  - In the **cycle of reactivity**, one person's limbic, fight-or-flight response triggers stress, self-doubt, and the fight-or-flight response in the other person. This reactivity in the second person then triggers more stress, self-doubt, and fight or flight in the first person, and so on, as shown in the figure below.

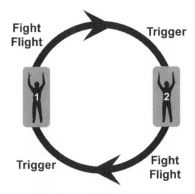

  - In contrast, the **cycle of creativity** is to give and receive love, as you mindfully engage with heart and mind, expressing yourself with authenticity and care, and listening with empathy and understanding.

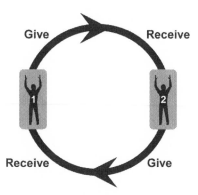

- Research also confirms the powerful effect of giving and receiving with empathy in the healthcare industry: a number of studies show that relationship-centered care and empathy affect a variety of patient outcomes, including patient satisfaction, reduction in physical pain, a positive response to psychotherapy, adherence to clinical advice, and even "business" outcomes such as patient retention, loyalty, and reduced malpractice risk.

- This cycle of creativity improves outcomes in business settings, too, as we'll discuss in more detail in chapter 11.

CHAPTER 10

Resolving Conflicts and Nurturing Your Relationships

The 4 in 4 Framework helps to facilitate the shift from reactivity to creativity anywhere along the relational spectrum—from resolving conflicts and finding agreement with the most difficult people in your life to nurturing all of your relationships, including those that bring you greatest joy.

Chapter 10, page 268

In chapter 10, you'll learn how to shift from cycles of reactivity to cycles of creativity in your relationships, whether at work or home. I begin by sharing the story of a coaching client, "Eric," an accomplished leader who had what he called a "horrendous" relationship with his son "Tony" and wanted to reconnect somehow. Within one year, after decades of intense reactivity, they were able to reunite, now more free to give and receive with each other in a cycle of creativity. What made the difference? Practicing the 4 in 4 Framework, specifically the four steps of Step 4.

Here you too will learn how to apply the four steps of Step 4 to mindfully give and receive in your relationships with kindness, empathy, and authenticity, allowing you to not only resolve your most reactive conflicts, but make your best relationships even better.

Key Points

- In chapter 8 (Step 4 of the 4 in 4 Framework), you learned how to use the Ask-Find-Evaluate-Apply cycle (see page 46 of this summary) to mindfully ask better questions; find, evaluate, and apply better answers; and therefore take more effective action. This process can help you make the shift from reactivity to creativity in your interactions with others as well and will be the key step in helping you **resolve conflict** and **nurture relationships**.

- To **resolve conflict** with the 4 in 4 Framework, begin by mindfully establishing your intention, or your "why," for resolving the conflict. Then consider how you can best *give* and *receive* by applying the four steps of Step 4:

  - ➤ First, **ask the right questions** to more clearly identify your conflict, identify the underlying triggers that may be driving it, and resolve your conflict. The first three steps can help frame your questions: for example, if you're experiencing strong reactivity, you may begin with questions that relate to Step 1, such as, "Am I limbic? Is the other person limbic? What are my sensations, thoughts, and feelings? Are my reactive responses causing the other person and me more harm than good?" For more examples of questions about giving and receiving based on Steps 1, 2, and 3 of the 4 in 4 Framework, see page 272.

  - ➤ Second, **find your answers.** One way to allow your answers to find you is to use a mindfulness practice to create a sense of loving-kindness for both yourself and the other person. (See page 274). From this place of greater stillness and clarity, you are better able to really listen to your intuition and find the answers that put you in the best possible position to heal the conflict.

  - ➤ Third, **evaluate your answers.** As you did in chapter 8, here you ask yourself, "Does this answer feel right more than feel good? Is this answer good for myself and others? Does this answer ultimately get me to a place where I am more likely to give and receive love?" (See page 275.)

  - ➤ Fourth, **apply your answers to take action.** This involves engaging in courageous communication to express yourself with care and deeply listen in to resolve your conflict. Further, it can be very helpful at the outset of your communication with the other person to set up rules of how you will give and receive with each other to provide you with the greatest likelihood of success. (See pages 276–278.)

> Finally, after you feel like you have applied most of your answers, you loop back to the first step by **asking questions again**. You might ask, "Are we now resolved?" or "Are we now in agreement?" When the answer is yes, and you've successfully taken action, you may experience an energy release, where the energy begins to flow in your relationship again. If the answer is no and you feel the conflict is still unresolved, or you are still holding on to energetic residue from your interaction, you return to your checklist of questions about receiving and giving from Step 1 and consider what other questions you can ask and actions you can take. (See pages 278-279.)

• To nurture your relationships at home and work, you can also use the four steps of Step 4 to mindfully give and receive.

> First, **ask the right questions**. For examples of specific questions about giving and receiving to nurture your relationships with family and friends, colleagues at work, clients or customers, patients (if you are a healthcare provider), and people you lead, see pages 281–286.

> Second, **find your answers** by taking some time to still yourself and allow the answers to find you. A simple and powerful way to do so is to imagine yourself breathing in the goodwill of others into your heart. Then you imagine yourself amplifying this feeling of goodwill in your heart and wishing them well by breathing out that goodwill into them. (See page 287.)

> Third, **evaluate your answers**. As in the resolving conflict section above, you again ask yourself, "Does this answer feel right more than feel good?"; "Is this answer good for myself and others?"; and ultimately, "Does this answer get me to a place where I am more likely to give and receive love?" (See page 287.)

> Fourth, **apply your answers to take action**. To be even more effective and present in doing so, here you learn how you can more mindfully take action. Just as you may focus on your breath in your mindfulness

breathing practice, here you can simply let the other person become your focus of attention to more fully nurture your relationships with them. (See pages 287–288.)

- A mindfulness practice that can further assist you in resolving conflicts and nurturing relationships is **Loving-Kindness (Part Two)**, which builds on the practice Loving-Kindness (Part One) you learned in chapter 6. For full instructions, see pages 288–291, or visit SuperSmartHealth.com/Book.

CHAPTER 11

Cultures of Reactivity and Creativity

The word culture comes from the Latin cultus, which means "care," and from the French colere, which means "to till," as in to till the ground. While the reactive mindset of low-performance leaders depletes the cultural soil of nourishment, causing people and their endeavors to wither, the creative mindset of high-performance (or conscious) leaders cultivates this soil, empowering people and allowing their endeavors to flourish.

Chapter 11, page 293

Just as our individual reactivity and creativity have a powerful effect on our relationships, leaders' reactivity and creativity are also socially contagious within cultures. In fact, it's been estimated that leaders determine 80 percent of the culture around them. And whether your culture is reactive or creative directly impacts your ability to create exceptional client experiences, and therefore your results. This is true whether you're the leader of a business, a nonprofit, a sports team, or a family.

In chapter 11, we connect the dots between leadership, culture, and profit. Then, in chapter 12, you'll learn how to apply the 4 in 4 Framework to your own culture, whether it's your business or other organization, your family, or your community.

Key Points

- As shown in the figure below, while leaders in a state of reactivity tend to trigger cycles and cultures of reactivity, creating negative client experiences and increasing cost, leaders in a state of creativity tend to trigger cycles and cultures of creativity, creating positive client experiences and increased profit.

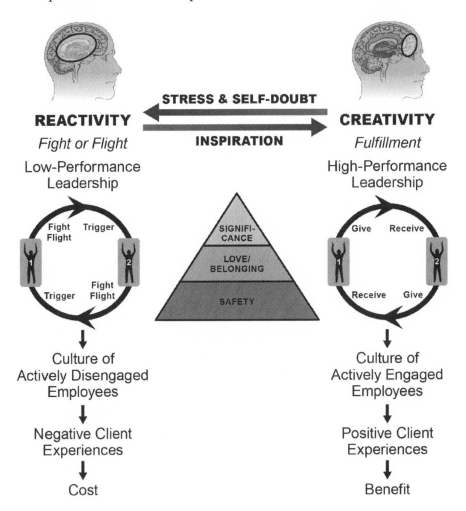

> Starting with the left side of the figure above, when a leader feels threatened by stress or self-doubt, they tend to go limbic, lose access to their circuits of empathy and compassion, and exhibit low-performance leadership behaviors. These behaviors trigger reactivity in their employees, which creates a self-perpetuating culture of threat and fear that unavoidably shows up on their faces and in their voices, erodes both morale and customer service, and results in a great cost to the company.

> On the right side of the figure, we see that a high-performance, creative leadership style creates the opposite results. High-performance leaders create cycles of giving and receiving in their relationships with employees, which is also socially contagious, creating a culture of actively engaged employees. As they are fully engaged in mind, heart, and soul, they become able to deliver exceptional hospitality and customer satisfaction, creating ever-expanding cycles of giving and receiving, which lead to profitable results.

> Both dynamics directly relate to Maslow's Hierarchy of Needs as well. While low-performance leaders threaten their employees' sense of safety and end up trapping them in survival mode at the bottom of the hierarchy, high-performance leaders facilitate the flow of energy all the way up Maslow's Hierarchy of Needs for each individual and the organization at large. They cultivate cultures where all experience safety and trust, love and belonging, and the ability to self-actualize their unique greatness and sense of significance.

- The chapter concludes with two powerful case studies epitomizing how creative, high-performing, Conscious Leaders pursuing their highest values have inspired thriving cultures of creativity.

CHAPTER 12

Transforming Families, Organizations, Communities, and the World

Leaders need to know how to sense and modulate the stress level of the culture to optimize the organization's energy and performance. In other words, they need to help increase and fully engage their company's resources to meet the demands they face. . . .

In this chapter, you'll learn how you can mindfully apply the 4 in 4 Framework to navigate stress at an organizational level and cultivate a high-performance culture of creativity and growth, whether it's at work, at home, or in your community.

Chapter 12, page 315

Now that you've learned how cultures of reactivity and creativity work, chapter 12 will help you cultivate a culture of creativity in your own context. Because the state of a leader is socially contagious, applying the 4 in 4 Framework in your groups as well as individually multiplies your positive impact as a leader.

Specifically, Chapter 12 shows you how to apply Steps 1–4 of the 4 in 4 Framework to the cultures you lead, whether it's a multinational corporation, healthcare facility, school, nonprofit, or family. You'll not only learn to help your culture navigate the threat of stress and cultivate a high-performance culture, but even help expand the peak performance potential of your organization!

Key Points

- Just as it does for individuals, the 4 in 4 Framework can empower you as a leader to facilitate the shift from a reactive to a creative culture.

  - To apply **Step 1: Recognizing and Managing Reactivity**, first identify any reactivity that may be present in your culture. For example, how prevalent is blame, gossip, judgment, bullying, or destructive conflict—or avoiding conflict with "artificial harmony"? You can also use validated instruments to evaluate your culture more formally. If you discover unhealthy reactivity, you can begin to manage it by adapting the four steps you learned in chapter 5: (1) pause, (2) breathe, (3) name it to tame it, and (4) consider your best response—which often leads you to Step 2. (See pages 316–318.)

  - To apply **Step 2: Reappraising Stress and Self-Doubt**, first, help your culture reappraise its collective mindset about stress and self-doubt. For example, you might share the research showing how you can leverage stress and self-doubt as assets. Then, rather than seeking to eliminate it, you can encourage people to engage more fully with what they care about most. Next, you can help identify and remove, wherever possible, the systematic triggers of stress that burden or constrain your environment. You can also adapt the four questions in the Appraise-Reappraise Method from chapter 6 (What happened?, What are our beliefs about what happened?, Are the beliefs really true?, and How can we view this differently?) to help defuse reactivity in a variety of contexts. (See pages 318–326.)

  - To apply **Step 3: Cultivate Creativity**, you can use the same VSIR Process you learned in chapter 7 for your organization. After clarifying your vision and mission, you next "look left before you turn right" and determine your SMART results and key performance indicators so you can track them. Then put your strategic plan in place, implement that strategy, and measure your results. If you miss your intended results, you then reiterate the cycle, reflecting on whether you need any changes in your vision, whether your strategy was comprehensive enough or if it was missing key components, where people fell short on implementation, or whether your results were realistic to begin with. You can then make ongoing changes as needed—in a cycle of continuous quality improvement—to collectively manifest your most meaningful vision, mission, and purpose. (See pages 326–334.)

> Culture can be thought of as the sum of all its conversations, both internal and external. To apply **Step 4: Catalyzing Growth**, you can use the Ask-Find-Evaluate-Apply cycle to facilitate more inspired internal and external dialogue in your organization, thus creating a more creative, growth-mindset culture. For example, at an inflection point instead of engaging shame-and-blame thinking about what's wrong with us or others, you can use this four-step cycle to engage in a more inspired internal dialogue. Ask mindful questions such as, "In this difficult moment, what are we here to learn?"; "How can we best connect with all our stakeholders?"; and "How can we express our best service?" With inspiring questions such as these, you can help your culture collectively shift from a threat response to a more adaptive challenge or tend-and-befriend response instead. (See pages 334–338.)

• Since living, breathing individuals (with their developing brains) make up living, breathing organizations, the peak performance curve shown on page 28 of this summary also represents the collective performance capacity of organizations. Thus, applying the steps of the 4 in 4 Framework within your organization may do more than help it achieve its peak performance. The new habits of thinking, beliefs, norms, and behaviors may create a collective neuroplastic transformation that shifts the performance curve up and to the right for the entire organization (see page 30 of this summary). This provides a neuroscience-based explanation of how companies can move from good to great!

• To further optimize your culture's energy and performance, you can use your own version of the mindfulness practice of **May We Serve Well Together**, which I used with the board of the Academy of Integrative Health and Medicine. For full instructions, see pages 340–342 in the book.

CONCLUSION

Lifelong Practice and Ongoing Transformation

Congratulations on becoming a more Conscious Leader!

You've come a long way. You've learned that conscious organizations with creative leaders perform better than others. The science proves it. And you've learned that if you want to create a more conscious organization or family or community, change has to start with you.

Conclusion, page 347

The key to your ongoing transformation is taking action. Research shows it takes about eight weeks to break old habits and create new ones. The good news is that as you continue to engage in the neuroscience- and mindfulness-based skills and practices of the 4 in 4 Framework, it will become easier and easier to leverage your stress and self-doubt into positive, productive energy and shift from a reactive, low-performance leadership state to a creative, high-performance leadership state in the heat of the moment. Over time, you'll also experience:

- Greater resilience

- More vibrant health

- Deeper relationships

- Greater success and significance at work and at home

I hope you have found this book summary helpful and that it has given you a solid sense of how the science and 4 in 4 Framework can benefit your personal life, your professional life, and the lives of those you lead.

I also hope it inspires you to immerse yourself further in the book itself. If you'd like to purchase the full version of *Leading Well from Within*, it's available at Amazon.com or at SuperSmartHealth.com/Book.

And if you'd like to dive into these principles and practices even more deeply, I would be honored to help you further develop and solidify your skills to lead well from within.

For individuals, SuperSmartHealth offers one-on-one coaching to deepen your learning and provide you with support to clarify and achieve the specific results you want for your life. We also offer online training and group coaching.

For organizations, we offer keynote speaking, live workshops, and executive coaching.

Just go to SuperSmartHealth.com to learn more.

I'd also welcome you to connect with me on:

LinkedIn: https://www.linkedin.com/in/danielfriedlandmd

Twitter: https://twitter.com/FriedlandMD

Facebook: https://www.facebook.com/supersmarthealth/

It is a joy and privilege to serve you.

With heartfelt appreciation,

Daniel

Daniel Friedland, MD

Dr. Daniel Friedland is an expert in the science of high-performance leadership.

He helps leaders and their organizations:

- Transform stress and burnout into resilience
- Make smarter health, business, and life decisions
- Optimize health, relationships, and productivity
- Thrive with greater meaning and purpose

Dr. Friedland wrote one of the first textbooks on Evidence-Based Medicine, which is the way healthcare providers are now trained to make science-based decisions. He is also the author of *The Big Decision*, which he wrote with his then-14-year-old son Zach, to inspire and empower better life decisions at home and at work.

An in-demand international expert in applying the framework of Evidence-Based Medicine to enhance decision-making, leadership, and resiliency, Dr. Friedland has worked with Fortune 500 companies; healthcare systems and medical groups; the US Army, Navy, and Air Force; Vistage; Young Presidents' Organization (YPO); Entrepreneurs' Organization (EO); The Global Wellness Summit; Conscious Capitalism; and leaders in the Texas and Australian governments. He's delivered over 1500 programs and presented to more than 75,000 healthcare and business professionals around the world.

Dr. Friedland is the founding chair of the Academy of Integrative Health and Medicine and the president and CEO of SuperSmartHealth, where he provides keynote addresses, live workshops, online programs, and executive coaching to cultivate Conscious Leadership.

"Dr. Danny" feels blessed to live in San Diego with his wife and two sons, where he gets to "surf his sympathetics" in the waves of California!

For more information about Dr. Danny and the programs, resources, and services he offers, please visit SuperSmartHealth.com.

Acknowledgments

Many thanks to Amanda Rooker, Executive Editor of SplitSeed, for her genius in editing my manuscript and helping at every stage of developing *Leading Well from Within*, including this book summary. Thanks also to Colin Webber for working on the cover design, Julie Felton for working further on the cover as well as the interior graphics, and Jay Polmar, Liliana Gonzalez Garcia, and the good people from iPublicidades for formatting the print and mobile versions of the book and summary. (Please see the book for expanded acknowledgments.)

Sue, I love and appreciate you and feel so blessed to be your partner. Thanks for your sage input on the book, this summary, and all you do to run our company—all enabling me to share this purposeful work. Zach and Dyl, I am deeply grateful to be your dad and love you both from the bottom of my heart.

I am humbled and deeply appreciative for the Source of inspiration that continues to inspire my life and this work, and has blessed me with my family and a purpose to share.

Finally, thanks to you for taking your valuable time to read this summary. I hope it inspires you to continue your journey of learning to lead well from within!